Return
to
Asylums

A Prescription for the American Mental Health System

Linda R Thompson, M.D.

Cover Design by Tami Barrett

The cover photo is of the Traverse Building taken from https://commons.wikimedia.org/wiki/File:Traverse,_Building_50.jpg. This is the Traverse City State Hospital from Traverse City, Michigan. The photo is in the public domain.

Table of Contents

Introduction

This report is in response to a viewpoint article by Dominic Sisti, PhD; Andrea G. Segal, MS and Ezekiel J. Emanuel, MD, PhD entitled "Improving Long Term Psychiatric Care: Bring Back the Asylum" that was published in *The Journal of the American Medical Association* (JAMA) in the January 20, 2015, issue.

I am likely one of the dwindling number of physicians and psychiatrists that have actually seen and worked on open wards and in state hospital settings. I was in medical school, internship and residency during the time the deinstitutionalization of the chronically mentally ill was moving into complete implementation in the 1960s. The open medical and surgical wards that I worked on during my internship were beginning to be phased out and replaced with private and semi-private rooms for inpatient care. I had enough experience with these open units in medicine as well as psychiatry to observe the efficiency and high quality of care that these units provided to the patients. The nursing station was located on the unit, giving the nursing staff continuous oversight of all the patients under their care. Patients' needs could be quickly identified and tended to very effectively.

The current system of care for the chronically mentally ill and also that for the severely mentally retarded is much less effective than the older style units. Some of the severely brain injured patients might also benefit from the older model of care. These patients are completely disabled by their psychosis, retardation or brain injury and will never be able to care for themselves without constant supervision and care. After reflecting on the experiences I had in my training years and my long-term work as a psychiatrist, I believe that a supportive long-term institution would provide the best care for these individuals. Additionally, it should be much more cost effective than our current system of care.

The possibility of returning to the asylum model can be easily rejected by well-meaning psychiatrists who have not seen what these older institutions can provide for these patients. I was motivated to write this report because it would be an unfortunate mistake to turn away from the recommendations that Dr. Sisti and his colleagues have made after careful research and consideration of all the options. Since I have had experience with the older system, I felt it was important to make this information available to those who will influence these decisions in the coming years.

Chapter One

A Deformed System

I had provided psychiatric services to several regional mental health centers for 30 years prior to my retirement from my consulting practice in August 2014, so I am very familiar with the services that are available for long-term outpatients in that setting. All of these centers had good administrators and good support for the staff. However, the services that they were able to offer were frequently defined by the financial incentives put in place by state and federal grants and by the services that private insurers, Medicare and Medicaid would reimburse. These services changed over time depending on what the latest thinking was among these larger agencies and insurers.

Sometimes services that were showing some benefit for the patients would be curtailed or discontinued due to changes in reimbursement. These decisions were not well informed medically. Because the budgets for providing services were always fairly tight, the centers had to adapt to the new standards, at times creating difficult transitions for patients.

Another issue that was frequently dictated by limited financial resources was the necessity of hiring recent graduates with very limited clinical experience as therapists or case managers. Often these individuals would move on to better positions or open a private practice after two or three years in the mental health center. The Department of Veterans Affairs (VA) Medical Center in our area was particularly prone to recruit our nurse practitioners after they had two or three years of experience under the supervision of the staff psychiatrists at the centers. They were able to do this by paying the practitioners much higher salaries than the mental health center could afford to pay. These situations created a significant turnover in staff which can be difficult for the long-term patients to deal with.

In addition to staffing challenges, insurance companies frequently pressured the psychiatric providers to change medications to the ones that were preferred on their formularies, even when patients had been stable on their current medications for several years. The insurance formularies could change on an annual basis, and that would automatically lead to required pre-authorizations for any medications no longer on the formulary. Getting pre-authorizations for the medications that were effective for a given patient became more and more time-consuming for the nursing staff. Over time we got fewer and fewer successful pre-authorizations. That meant that the patient had to try and fail two of the insurers' drugs before being allowed to return to their original medication.

All of these financial and staff constraints impacted the care of the patients in significant and unavoidable ways. Starting over with a new therapist or psychiatrist was difficult when the patient had developed a good therapeutic relationship with the provider who was leaving. The mandated changes in medications dictated by the insurance companies also created instability in the patient's long-term care that could sometimes lead to a relapse of their illness and/or to medication non-compliance. Any negative outcomes would of course be blamed on the patient and/or the provider.

This is just a brief summary of the issues that impact the consistency of outpatient care and support for these long term patients. For the more psychotic, paranoid and unstable of these patients, these inconsistencies make it almost impossible for them to get into long-term outpatient treatment. And should they require emergency involuntary hospitalization, the commitment process (covered in the fourth chapter in this report) is difficult enough to leave them even more paranoid about the system as a whole.

These limitations make it increasingly difficult to provide the consistency necessary to build trust with this very vulnerable and challenged population.

It is naive to think that there would be enough funding available to correct these problems to an extent that would make the system workable for these patients. It would require them to be higher functioning and less paranoid than their illnesses allow.

I have a lot of respect for the mental health centers and what they accomplish with higher functioning patients with serious mental illness despite the administrative challenges they face. However, rather than trying to find a way to fit these very unstable patients into this system, it seems more realistic to utilize the extensive experience of the senior mental health center staff as a resource for helping develop long-term institutions for the chronically mentally ill.

I believe the word deformation could be very appropriately applied to this current medical system. We are now working in a professional system that has been literally deformed by financially driven decisions that have been to the detriment of our patients. Medicine is a profession. Business issues have to be addressed if one is to earn a living in this profession. However, running a practice primarily as a business and only secondarily as a profession will provide little satisfaction to the ethical practitioner and poorer outcomes to our patients.

Rather than continue to try to find a way to serve these much less stable patients in this malfunctioning system, I must agree with Dr. Sisti and his co-authors in their call for the return to the long-term institutions. The issue of asylums is simply one instance of a larger problem in medicine: how to find a way to take ethical and professional care of our patients in a seriously dysfunctional system. And it is one whose time has come again.

I hope this report will add to the conversation that Dr. Sisti and his group initiated in their JAMA opinion piece in January 2015 and provide a broader context for beginning to address the deformation and dysfunction that we as physicians and psychiatrists see every day in our work with patients.

Chapter Two

Adults In Need of Asylum Care

"Return to Asylums? Never!" was the demonstrative title of the "From the President" column in the August 21, 2015, issue of the *Psychiatric News*, the newspaper of the American Psychiatric Association (APA). Renee Binder, MD, then president of the APA, reported on her debate with Dominic Sisti, PhD, a medical ethicist who had proposed a return to asylums. The debate took place at the Commonwealth Club of California, the nation's oldest and largest public affairs forum. Dr. Sisti argued that a return to asylums was the most ethical solution to the current problem of inadequate care for the chronically mentally ill.

Many of the population in question are currently psychotic and living a very precarious life of homelessness with occasional acute hospitalization for severe psychotic episodes. If they have family support, they may be able to make use of community resources for treatment of their ongoing and frequently treatment-resistant psychotic illnesses. However, many of these families are overwhelmed by the needs of these patients. Relatives may also be legitimately afraid of them, since they may be intermittently very paranoid and pose a risk of harm to others. Unfortunately, for now the only institution that can provide long-term institutional care for them is the prison system, which already houses a significant percentage of these chronically ill individuals. We are now back to the conditions of the 1840s when there were more mentally ill persons in jails and prisons than in hospitals according to a report entitled *More Mentally Ill Persons Are in Jails and Prisons Than Hospitals: A Survey of the States* (Torrey, Kennard, Eslinger, Lamb, & Pavle,

2010). They additionally indicated that "40 percent of individuals with serious mental illnesses have been in jail or prison at some time in their lives" (Torrey, et al., 2010).

Dr. Binder acknowledged the current problems that these patients have in trying to live within the community but recommended the development of additional community resources for them. She sees the goal of such programs as the fostering of independence and autonomy in these individuals. Conversely, she sees asylums as an avenue toward *de*pendence, to an infantilized existence in state care.

Contrary to Dr. Binder's opinion, it has been my experience with acutely ill schizophrenic patients, that if they fail to respond to medication within a short period of time, they already begin to show the negative symptoms of schizophrenia. Common symptoms include flat affect, isolation from others, inattention to the normal activities of daily life and a general inability to deal with ordinary levels of stress without becoming overwhelmed, agitated and/ or more psychotic. In these instances the symptoms are not caused by long-term institutional care because this option has not existed for many years.

The President's unit at St. Elizabeth's Hospital in Washington, DC is probably the only long-term unit of this sort still in existence. And it will remain in existence because the patients in that unit are considered to be threats to the president and in need of life-long inpatient treatment. John Hinckley, the man who shot President Reagan in an assassination attempt, is the best known of these residents.

I have had the experience of observing the long-term care provided to these patients in the old asylums while I was in my residency in psychiatry in the late 1960s. I was in the residency program at the University of Virginia (UVA) Hospital in Charlottesville, Virginia from 1967 through 1971. The closest of the asylums in Virginia was Western State Hospital in Staunton, and I was able to observe the patients in that setting on several occasions.

I was also on the resident staff at the UVA Hospital Department of Psychiatry Mental Health Center. Some of the patients who were being discharged from Western State came to the center for treatment. It was very difficult to get them stabilized in the community setting, particularly those who had been institutionalized for 15 or 20 years. In a number of instances they no longer had living relatives to take them in when they were released from the asylum. I knew of at least one suicide in this patient group during the six months of my mental health center rotation. Some patients could not be released at all due to the fact that their condition appeared to represent a risk to members of the community to which they would return.

By the end of my residency, I was convinced that the idea that the long-term hospitals were the cause of negative symptoms of schizophrenia or chronic manic-depressive illness was simply wrong. Even now, after more than 50 years of general psychiatric practice, I have not changed my mind about this issue. I firmly believe that the asylums are the most ethical and humane setting in which to care for these individuals. It makes no sense to blame the institutions for the dependency needs of these patients. These needs are simply another aspect of their devastating illnesses.

These are severely debilitating illnesses and frequently treatment-resistant. They leave these patients significantly disabled and no longer capable of autonomy. Young males with this level of illness in particular have a very poor prognosis. These patients became the ones who would sit in the day room on our ward, frequently rocking back and forth and looking at others with empty eyes. We had a term for those with that look: a "burned out schizophrenic."

The availability of psychotropic medications has spared many milder schizophrenic patients from this level of dependence. But for those patients who remain chronically psychotic in spite of appropriate treatments, they have simply lost the capacity to return to a more independent state. In this instance, they are more like individuals who have suffered a severe brain injury. They will never return to their previous level of functioning.

One young man tragically typified this state. He was eighteen or nineteen years old and was very delusional when he was brought to the hospital. He believed that someone had taken his head and replaced it with a new head that did not work right. He spent his days and many nights as well, wandering the unit searching for his old head. This behavior did not change with any of the medications that we tried. And while his delusion was psychotic in that no one had really taken his head, it was also a poignant description of what this devastating illness had done to his mind.

Unfortunately, many of the buildings that housed these long-term patients have now been torn down or simply neglected for many years, making them unfit for use at this point. When I first went into practice after completing my residency, I worked for six months at the Northern Virginia Mental Health Institute, which was a new state hospital in Fairfax, Virginia, built to provide acute and subacute care to seriously mentally ill individuals. It was more like the regular psychiatric units at the University of Virginia Hospital and bore little resemblance to the typical asylum units at Western State Hospital. Once patients at the Northern Virginia Mental Health Institute had exhausted their insurance benefits and could no longer pay for continued treatment at that hospital, they would be transferred to Western State, which had always taken medically indigent patients from northern and western Virginia. The patients who would be transferred to Western State were the typical patients who required long-term institutional care.

One of the positive aspects of these longer-term treatment institutions that I have not seen mentioned in many years, is that of the staff situations in these facilities. In many instances, the staffing had been provided by second, third and even fourth generations of family members, who had been committed to the care of these patients over multiple generations. This was an invaluable asset to the institutions and a dedicated calling for the families who maintained that relationship to these patients. While the value of these committed and skilled staff members could not be measured in terms of monetary wealth, this would be an excellent example of social capital which has now been lost with the deinstitutionalization movement. It will not be easily renewed, even if the asylums were to be reopened for these patients tomorrow.

Because of this long-term continuity, the staff was very familiar with their patients, enough to determine which were safe to allow off-unit during the day and which, because of unpredictability and/or violent tendencies, needed to be contained in the unit. They would selectively allow some patients the freedom to move around the buildings and grounds of the institution, sometimes even allowing them to help out in the gardens that were maintained on the grounds. These gardens provided some of the food for the patients as well as the on-duty staff.

I was able to observe the compassionate care the nursing staff provided for a 25-year-old woman, who had a very early and very devastating onset of Huntington's chorea, which resulted in her being placed at Western State Hospital. Chorea is the name for abnormal involuntary writhing movements of the body, and Huntington's Disease, as it is now called is the most common cause of these movements. In the later stages of the illness, the movements become more violent, and patients can be thrown through windows or abruptly onto the floor, causing very serious injuries that can even be life-threatening. In addition to the involuntary movements, these patients typically become demented as the disease progresses. This illness is a genetically determined disease, and the gene that causes the disorder is an autosomal dominant gene. This means that each child born to a carrier parent has a 50% chance of inheriting the disorder. Since genetic testing has become available, many of the carriers have been identified and have chosen not to have children. The usual late onset of the disease in the patient's 40s or 50s, meant that there could already be children in the family who were at risk of the disease. There is no known cure for this illness.

This young woman was demented by the time I saw her and was in restraints to prevent her being thrown abruptly from her bed by the severe and violent chorea-form movements that accompanied her illness. This patient was heavily sedated to keep her as comfortable as possible. She had a cast on her left arm from a recent fall that had fractured her wrist and forearm. I do not know whether she had living family or not, but she clearly could not be managed in any other setting. The continual deteriorating course of her neurodegenerative disease required full-time care that was only available in a long-term medical institution. Patients such as this could not be managed in the typical nursing home.

I also saw several patients in classic catatonic states, mostly bedridden in the unit. Catatonia is one of the more serious symptoms of schizophrenia and manic depressive illness. The patient appears stuporous and unresponsive. He or she may remain in the same position for hours without moving. If someone positions their arm, for instance, in an elevated or outstretched position, the patient will maintain this position for hours. Catatonia is also associated with other illnesses as well, including some neurological illnesses. It is sometimes secondary to medication effects. Patients in this state require complete physical care.

There were at least 50 to 75 beds in an open ward. There were separate wards for male and female patients. The nursing station was mid-way down the length of the unit and open to the ward. The staff appeared to know all the patients very well. They were alert to changes in a patient's demeanor or behavior that would signal trouble. They were quick to intervene to avoid the situation escalating, and they did so calmly but firmly. If this was not successful, a male orderly would take the threatening patient to one of the seclusion rooms and spend some time with him or her until he or she was calm enough to return to the unit. There was always a male nursing assistant on every shift in the event one of the patients had to be physically restrained. If a patient needed a longer time in seclusion, the patient would remain in seclusion. He or she would be given additional medication to help them stabilize and to treat agitation if that was part of the issue.

I did not spend a lot of time in these units, but I never saw the staff mistreat any of the patients when he or she was agitated and out of control. The staff maintained a safe environment, and the patients were generally accepting of the interventions of the nurses when these became necessary. One of my sisters completed three months at one of the Virginia state hospitals for her psychiatric training as a nursing student. She also reported that the patients received good care in the institution. She had seen no evidence of abuse.

Most of the patients had a flat affect and appeared apathetic much of the time. The unit environment was a low-stimulus setting that did not make any demands on the patients. The routine of activities was the same from one day to the next, and the schedule of meals, tidying, bedtime, etc. was very predictable. This provided a therapeutic, benign structure for the patients, one they generally were incapable of providing for themselves. They benefited from the structure and were at a loss as to how to organize their lives if they were discharged from the asylum.

If the discharged patients were living independently, they generally did not maintain their hygiene or clean their rooms or apartments without prompting. They usually had little interaction with neighbors or other members of the community. If they were stable in treatment and compliant with their medications, they could exist in the community setting. However they usually remained isolated except for contact with doctors, therapists, case managers and with family members if they were available.

There is a fairly high incidence of alcohol, drug and nicotine abuse in these patients. One study in the US found 47% of patients had some substance abuse issues at some time during the course of their illness (Buckley, Miller, Lehrer, & Castle, 2009). The substance abuse will usually interfere with the patient getting optimal benefit from medication. Without someone checking on them fairly frequently, they deteriorate, generally becoming noncompliant with medication and then further descending into homelessness and/or illegal activities, which can lead to hospitalization or incarceration. Further complicating matters, while they are homeless, they are easily preyed upon by more aggressive or exploitive persons.

The notion that some of these patients could be managed in nursing homes as they get older now seems to be coming into question. There was a story recently in the local newspaper, reported from New York, that described how nursing homes are turning to eviction as a way of coping with their most difficult and challenging residents ("Nursing homes turn to eviction to drop difficult patients," Associated Press, May, 2016). Many of those chosen for evictions are poor and demented. They are generally difficult to manage behaviorally and require a lot of staff time to keep things manageable for them and the other residents. Families have a very difficult time finding another placement for them, and any change in their residence is generally very disorganizing for these vulnerable individuals. Federal data from the Long-Term Care Ombudsman Program reported 11,331 grievances filed in 2014 related to instances of evictions or attempted evictions from adult-care settings (Nursing homes, 2016). To put that in perspective, there were approximately 1,383,000 nursing home residents in the United States on December 31, 2012 according to a report from the Department of Health and Human Services entitled *Nursing Home Data Compendium 2013 Edition..* Of that number, 15% or 207,450 were under 65, leaving 1,175,550 residents who are 65 or older.

There are groups who are attempting to block such evictions as very harmful to the individuals evicted. On the other hand, the American Healthcare Association, which represents nursing homes, cites issues of safety as a reasonable justification for such involuntary discharges. They point to instances where the staff is unable to guarantee the safety of the person and/ or the safety of other residents of the facility (Nursing homes, 2016). These patients are seen as needing a level of care that goes beyond what the typical nursing home can offer. Long-term care in an asylum setting would probably be a better solution for these very difficult patients. And the ready availability of psychiatric treatments would be an additional asset to their care.

Chapter Three

Children in Need of Asylum Care

While my early practice focused on adults for the most part (perhaps 30% of my practice was children then), for the past 12 years I have worked almost exclusively with children and adolescents. In that capacity I have seen a number of pediatric patients who needed a level of care on par with that of the adults in the last chapter. They too would have benefitted from the low stimulus environment an institution can provide.

The families and school systems are overwhelmed and even endangered by the extreme needs of these children. Some of these pediatric patients have severe psychiatric illnesses that can be as treatment-resistant as those we see in the adult chronically ill population. Other children have suffered severe early trauma that has left them violent and with no capacity for meaningful relationships. Autistic children commonly become agitated and/or violent if something in the immediate environment overwhelms them. Special education classes, while providing a respite for exhausted parents and some appropriate developmental stimulation for the pupils, are not the best place for these severely mentally impaired students any more than a regular community is a good fit for a severely impaired adult.

One of the autistic boys that I saw for seven or eight years would become violent if he was overwhelmed. It was not always clear what had set him off, as he was almost completely non-verbal. At times he would take off his clothes in the classroom and would strike out at the teachers and aides who were trying to keep him clothed. When he was really out of control, he would smear his bowel movements on the walls, the floor or sometimes on the staff or other students.

By the time he was in high school, he was almost six feet tall and weighed about 240 pounds. When he became violent, he was a serious danger to the teaching staff as well as the other students. After several difficult episodes with him in the school setting, the school would put him on homebound status. Dismissal from school left his mother, who was a single parent, to care for a sometimes violent and uncooperative "child" who was six inches taller and 50 pounds heavier than she was, a recipe for disaster. She had full time responsibility for his care when he was not in school, and he was a danger to her when he became violent. His grandfather tried to help his mother and had some early success with him. The boy sometimes stayed with his grandfather to give his mother a break from the constant demands of his care. During the last year he was at home, however, he would sometimes become violent with his grandfather also.

His behavior would typically continue to spiral down while home-bound, necessitating large doses of a number of antipsychotic and mood stabilizing medications. At times even this treatment would prove inadequate for his needs. He was hospitalized twice in a special unit in middle Tennessee that accepted him with his diagnosis of autism. He would stabilize while there, but his negative behaviors would resurface when he returned home again. Clearly the atmosphere of the institution played a large part in the successful treatment of this young patient. Unfortunately it was not a long-term option.

Once he was eighteen, his mother lost even the respite of his intermittent public school attendance, and because of his tendency toward violent behavior, he was refused at every available treatment facility. Desperate, exhausted, and endangered, his mother turned to a family friend whose significant political influence finally secured long-term residential care for this troubled young man.

I have treated several other boys, with illnesses ranging from bipolar disorder to conduct disorder, from autism to childhood psychosis, who were also prone to violence when upset. The family members who are their primary caretakers are endangered by continued assaults when the boys are out of control. These behaviors are usually manageable when they are very young. But as they grow, the assaults become harder to deal with. Most of them have had placements at residential treatment centers for several months up to a year. They have had minimal, if any, improvement during their placements, and they remain a danger to their family when they return home. Most of these boys are now well into adolescence and have a lot of physical strength making them more dangerous when they lose control.

I saw one boy who was in the custody of his grandparents from a young age. He had been physically abusive at times toward his grandmother, and this became worse as he entered puberty. His grandfather had been able to maintain control of him by setting very firm limits. Once he was adolescent, he became more verbally defiant with his grandfather, and he began to threaten violence. He had one residential placement of several months duration while still in middle school. It appeared likely that he would need another placement while in high school. I prescribed large doses of anti-psychotic and mood stabilizing medicines without success, and the medications prescribed at the residential placement did not stabilize his condition either. I was concerned that he would seriously injure his grandmother in one of his rages and possibly his grandfather as well. He had an intensive in-home case manager that worked with him and his grandparents on a weekly basis. They had safety plans in place and could call 911 for help if necessary. His grandparents had decided that if his behavior became consistently uncontrollable, they would not continue to provide care for him.

This boy had poor social skills and was almost constantly intimidating others in an attempt to get his way. He was mildly mentally challenged, making little academic progress in his special education classes. He was not going to be able to live independently when he finished school. Most likely he would end up in a correctional facility since his level of violence would make any other placement very unlikely. This would not be an ideal outcome for him but would keep him from harming others in the community. I believe a long-term institutional placement would be a much more appropriate solution for this young man and the others like him.

Grandparents are raising quite a few of these boys, inheriting their custody after their removal from chaotic early home environments, frequently involving abuse and neglect. Some of them also had in vitro exposure to alcohol and/or drugs. Each form of these early traumas creates additional risks of violent behaviors that pose a threat of harm to others. In Tennessee they can continue in public school until they are twenty-two years old, which gives their caretakers a break, but this is not available for them if they are a danger to other students or school staff. Because violence is an issue with these patients, they will most likely be institutionalized in the prison setting at some point, since their history of violence renders them ineligible for treatment at most psychiatric units.

Though the boys have a higher tendency toward violence, I have seen a few girls who were also prone to dangerous outbursts and equally difficult to treat. I treated one such young girl who was the oldest child in a family with three children. She was nonverbal and thought to have some kind of rare genetic disorder. She had been tested for several possibilities without success. She did not respond to any of the different prescribed medications and continued to have frequent behavioral outbursts. She was occasionally violent with her younger siblings, and she would also hit, kick and bite her parents when she was angry. These behaviors continued at school where she would accost classmates and teachers, as well as their aides. She was profoundly retarded. The parents were struggling to give the two younger children as normal a childhood as they possibly could. However, keeping this child from disrupting the home environment took almost all the resources this family had. When I last saw her, she was about eight years old and had had no response to any treatments offered over a three or four year duration of care. Like the violent young men described above, an institutional placement, had it been available, would have been the most appropriate setting for the care of this patient with her very specialized needs.

Violent outbursts happen more frequently without the firm leadership of a healthy, strong, engaged adult. With custodial care so frequently defaulting to aging grandparents, a new complication therefore arises. Whereas parents would have been able to tend to the troubled children well into that child's adulthood, a custodial grandparent will offer 20 to 30 fewer years of effective care for the troubled grandchildren. This is even shorter in the rare instances that a great grandparent becomes the custodial parent for one of these children. And I have treated three children who were being reared by great-grandparents, in two instances by single parent great-grandmothers. Violent tendencies in the absence of a strong parental advocate lead inevitably to the criminal justice system.

Having a benign institutional placement for children like this would seem to be a better intervention than trying to keep them stabilized in the family and the public school system. And it could give them much more appropriate care than the correctional system would be able to. There is currently no such placement available for these children. The development of such facilities would require a major rethinking of the psychiatric treatments for severely impaired and chronically mentally ill patients of all ages.

An issue that was not addressed in the Binder/Sisti debate was the use of asylums or long-term institutions for mentally handicapped (now termed mentally challenged) individuals. There were state institutions that were devoted to the life-long care of these individuals. In my third year of medical school in the fall of 1964, I visited one such institution, the Lynchburg Colony in Lynchburg, Virginia.

The institution took in newborn babies with Down's syndrome, severe brain damage and other congenital malformations that would result in profound mental retardation. Severely physically disabled children with mental impairment could also be placed in these facilities. Families could choose to keep their child or turn the child over to state custody following their birth.

At the Lynchburg Colony there was an infant's nursery of 8 to 10 cribs for the children who were not yet walking. Additionally, there was a toddler's room with 10 to 15 beds. The toddlers also had a playroom where they were allowed to play freely. They were not at all bothered by our group of strangers. Most of them were Down's syndrome children and they were very willing to interact with us briefly before they lost interest and went back to play with the other children. Their lack of identifying us as a group of strangers was a result of their limited cognitive abilities.

The children appeared to be kept with their age-mates throughout their early childhood. At some point, probably before adolescence, they were segregated by gender and kept in same sex units. When they were 18 to 20 years old, they were then moved onto one of the adult units where they remained for the rest of their lives.

In most instances the families chose to forgo a relationship with these children once they were placed in state care. However, I know of one instance of a family who maintained a relationship with their son while he was a residential ward of the state. He had been diagnosed with severe mental retardation after appearing to be healthy at birth. He became brain-damaged due to a genetic disease called phenylketonuria (PKU). His body was unable to break down the amino acid phenylalanine, which unfortunately is in most of the foods in the usual American diet. He built up a toxic level of this amino acid in his body, and this toxicity interfered with the development of his brain. Tragically it was too late to undo the damage, and his parents placed him at the Lynchburg Colony when he was three or four years old. They still visited him once or twice a month and were able to take him out in the town for several hours before taking him back to the institution. The staff welcomed them when they visited, and their continued relationship with their son was clearly respected by the staff and the administration.

Some time later, just as it became popular to transition the chronically mentally ill out of facilities and into their communities of origin, there was also a shift in the expectations of parents of severely mentally handicapped children. Families were generally expected to care for their severally disabled children. Where the families were unable to take on the responsibility of caring for such a damaged child, the state would place these children in foster care instead of residential treatment and, if possible, allow them to be adopted into families willing to care for them.

I have provided psychiatric services to some of these children during the past 32 years of my general psychiatric practice. Some of these patients would have been served far more effectively in a long-term residential facility. The institution that served these mentally handicapped individuals in northeast Tennessee was called Green Valley Development Center. It had been slowly reducing the number of residents in the institution over the previous 15 to 20 years and was finally closed down around the time that I was leaving my consulting position at Frontier Health-Bristol Regional Counseling Center in August of 2014.

It is unclear at this point how these mentally challenged individuals will be cared for over the long-term since they will always require care and close supervision throughout their lives. They will never be independent or self-sufficient. As their parents become too old or disabled to care for them, there is no longer an institution available to take over their care for the remainder of their lives.

I am very concerned about the problems in the long term care of these individuals. I am distressed that a very functional and humane system of care for these patients has been systematically dismantled and destroyed over the past 40 years, seemingly in the interests of giving these individuals a more personalized level of care. However, this supposed better level of care has failed to materialize for many of them.

One of the goals was to promote improved self-sufficiency and independence in these people. This is a very unrealistic goal for most of them. It is also a very expensive and unsustainable way to provide care for them. This is one of the reasons that the United States has the highest healthcare costs in the world. It would be wise to look closer at the work done by Dr. Sisti and his colleagues at the University of Pennsylvania. It would be especially interesting to see if they have addressed the economic issues of a transition back to an earlier, yet more practical form of care for these patients.

Chapter Four

Descent into Deinstitutionalization

The asylum system of care I've described didn't just spring up one day any more than it disappeared overnight. It was intentional, a response to a demonstrated need. It had grown out of the work of people like Dorothea Dix, an American activist for the indigent and insane starting in the mid-1830s while she was in England. She spent some time with a group of English people who were advocating for "Lunacy Reform," as it was called in England. She returned to America and began to investigate the conditions of asylums in the Boston area in 1840 and 1841. This led to a report that she wrote for the Massachusetts legislature, outlining the deplorable conditions that many of these mentally ill individuals suffered. She continued to work for improvement in the care of these psychiatrically ill individuals throughout several states in the 1840s and 1850s. Her work greatly influenced and improved the treatment of the mentally ill in many of these states, leading ultimately to the establishment of a number of state-financed and state-run institutions for the care of these patients.

So why did something so effective fall out of favor? There appear to be a number of issues that led to the movement to deinstitutionalize these patients in the late 1950s and early 1960s. One of them was the reports of abusive treatment of these patients in some of the state institutions, particularly Massachusetts' Bridgewater State Hospital which generated public support for finding better solutions for the care of these patients. There were charges that patients were simply being warehoused in these institutions without being provided with treatments that would allow them to recover. The institutions were also blamed for the negative symptoms of schizophrenia, stating that they were a direct result of the deprivations the patients suffered in the institutions. As I have discussed in previous chapters, this was in fact an erroneous assumption.

Also contributing to mass deinstitutionalization was the development of multiple psychotropic medications that effectively treated many of these individuals, occasionally with even full remission of most of their psychotic symptoms. They were then better able to leave the asylums, managing residual symptoms in an outpatient setting. This revolutionized the practice of psychiatry. Many people were spared the experience of being in an institution and were able to become functioning members of their local communities.

Advancements in pharmaceuticals would affect the existence of long-term medical facilities in another way: they would bring about the closure of all the tuberculosis sanitariums. These sanitariums were government-funded hospitals for the mandatory quarantining and treatment of all identified patients with active tuberculosis. There were no exceptions made for these patients; they were immediately sent to the sanitarium as soon as they were diagnosed. They were then held there until their disease became inactive or they died. While these patients were not psychiatric patients, the facilities themselves- had they not been closed- could have provided appropriate space for some of the patients discussed herein.

As much as public opinion and the pharmaceutical industry moved our country away from the asylum system, the almighty dollar was the nail in the proverbial coffin of what was once an effective design. These institutions were initially established when there were enough wealthy patients (American and otherwise) who could afford to pay out-of-pocket for their treatment. The increases in coverage for psychiatric illnesses in the 1950s and 1960s, mostly in federal insurance plans, opened up the possibility for many middle class individuals to obtain treatment for their mental illnesses. The availability of this coverage was an outgrowth of the expanding and prosperous economy of the US during that time. Unfortunately, we are no longer in an expanding economy, and the resources to pay for the care of these individuals are becoming more and more strained. The rise and fall of the asylum system closely follows that of the US economy.

In the mid-1960s, President Lyndon Johnson's Great Society plan included Medicare, Medicaid, a War on Poverty, etc., and all these things were readily funded because of their popularity. As the decade and Johnson's term drew to a close, the collective national mindset was turning and has yet to come full circle.

The passing of the Medicare Act of 1965 gave individual insurance benefits to the indigent and elderly. Social Security gave psychiatric patients an opportunity to have disability income, which also afforded them the opportunity to live somewhat independently, even if they did not have a family to whom they might return. Community mental health centers were developed at this time to allow people to get quality outpatient psychiatric care in their home communities. This was initially funded by federal and state grant money as part of the commitment to deinstitutionalize these patients. It was assumed that with the new medications and new outpatient mental health centers that these people would be able to live somewhat normal lives once they were deinstitutionalized. But not every patient's mental illness is treatable with pharmaceuticals, and healthcare benefits have taken quite a journey since the 1960s.

In the 1960s, federal insurance plans covered the cost of psychiatric illnesses, allowing a full year for inpatient treatment and generous outpatient services as well. Some of the larger corporate insurances would provide 120 days of inpatient treatment for employees and their families. Quite a few government employees were able to get full psychoanalytic treatment through the major medical part of their federal insurance. There were long-term hospitals for those requiring inpatient treatment in many urban areas, and the hospitals became dependent on the insurance coverage for more and more of their patients.

Starting in the mid 1970s, however, the insurers (including those who provided coverage through the federal plans) began to curtail the benefits available for psychiatric inpatient as well as outpatient treatments. This led to the closure of many of these treatment centers. Two of these surviving institutions, McLean Hospital in Boston and Shepphard Pratt Health System in Baltimore have now reopened long-term inpatient treatment programs that are not funded by insurance. But this makes them available only to the wealthier patients who can pay out-of-pocket for their care.

Beginning in the 1990s, getting authorization for even a two or three week inpatient stay became more and more difficult. Today when someone is hospitalized in a psychiatric unit, their length of stay depends on the insurer's determination of continued inpatient treatment as "medically necessary", and the authorizations are done on an almost daily basis. Even with medication treatments, the patients are discharged to outpatient treatment within 10 days on average. This is several weeks before the medication will have either reached full benefit or failed to provide an adequate response. Psychiatrists and other mental health workers are expected to assess the patient's risk for harm to self and others and provide effective treatment within a very short period of time, seven to ten days in most instances. This is wishful thinking at its worst and leads to discharges that are seriously premature in many instances. And recent changes in insurance guidelines for medical hospitalizations penalize the hospital by denying additional reimbursement if a patient is readmitted to the hospital for the same problem within a set number of days (30-90, depending on the insurance company). I expect this to be done with psychiatric hospitalizations also if it hasn't already. This will significantly increase the risks for many patients as well as providers.

Psychiatrists are no longer even allowed to use their professionally trained discretion to commit a patient directly to a psychiatric unit, but rather must refer the patient and responsible family members to their closest emergency room to be evaluated by a crisis worker. This individual assesses the patient, and if they determine there is justification, they get initial approval from the patient's insurer and find a local or regional hospital that will take the patient. The patient and family members may spend up to 10 hours waiting to see the crisis worker. This delay sometimes temporarily calms the patient, resulting in a refusal of admission by the crisis worker. But the patient who is truly in need of inpatient care will shortly return to an unstable state, prompting a repeat of this lengthy, exhausting, unproductive procedure- sometimes multiple times- before an admission is finally completed.

On several occasions, in order to ensure the safety of all involved, I have even advised the parents of a dangerously out of control adolescent patient to refuse to take the patient home on the grounds that they do not feel safe doing so. In these instances the patient remains in the ER long enough to become violent or threatening, and then the emergency room staff has to bring in one or more security guards to stay with the patient until hospitalization can be arranged. In one instance the patient remained under guard in the emergency room for four days before an admission was finally accomplished.

There have also been times when adult patients remain in the emergency room under guard and awaiting involuntary admission sometimes for as long as several weeks. In some of these instances, the patient will improve enough that he or she will be discharged from the emergency room to outpatient treatment. If the patient remains a risk for harming self or others they will eventually be hospitalized. These patients will be transported to the hospital by the local sheriff's office, and many times they will go in handcuffs in the back of the deputy's car as if they had committed some crime. And because we lack the long term facilities to appropriately treat these patients, many wind up in the back of the deputy's car because they *have* committed a crime.

In fact, the current climate has left the penal system to care for a large number of these patients. According to the Bureau of Justice Statistics, over half of all prisoners in 2005 had experienced mental illness. Of this population, 60% of jail inmates had psychiatric symptoms, while 49% of state inmates and 40% of federal prisoners were symptomatic (James & Glaze, 2006). The percentage of those prisoners who had a recent history of mental illness was 21% for jail inmates, 24% for state prisoners and 14% for those in federal prisons (James et al., 2006). To put this in perspective, according to the US Bureau of Justice Statistics (BJS) there were a total of 2,220,300 prisoners in state and federal prisons and in local jails at the end of 2013.

With the escalation of violence in the nation and the need to provide containment for people who are at risk of violent assaults on others, it is frustrating that our mental health system is more and more hampered by the rules and regulations of non-medically trained individuals. These people are employed by and therefore beholden to the insurance companies and other systems, including certifying agencies, large for-profit healthcare corporations, corrections institutions and private prison corporations. Their policies and procedures can negatively impact these individuals' ability to obtain treatment when they are at their most vulnerable. Many of the most dangerous are already paranoid and distrustful of the mental health system, and this is an additional hindrance to getting them actively engaged in a therapeutic process.

What began as a well-intentioned program, with an earnest desire to help those who desperately need it, has become a victim of multiple, largely economic policies. This is a broken system and inadequate for meeting the patient's legitimate needs for treatment in a timely manner and with a realistic length of stay. We need to undo deinstitutionalization. We need to REinstitutionalize.

Chapter Five

Recovery Needs

Dr. Sisti's 2015 viewpoint piece reports that in 1955, the United States had 560,000 long-term psychiatric patients in state-run facilities. He goes on to state that there are currently 45,000 patients in state psychiatric facilities (Sisti, et al., 2015). I do not know the location of a single state facility in Tennessee or Virginia that provides long-term care. The hospitals I am familiar with provide acute and subacute care with a somewhat longer length of stay than private psychiatric units, but this is longer by only a few weeks.

I have recently learned about the Asylum Projects, which is a Wikipedia undertaking, that has a significant amount of information on the past history and current status of the older asylums in all fifty states plus Puerto Rico and the District of Columbia. Their website is www.asylumprojects.org.

Private psychiatric hospital beds are mostly for acute care now, and the length of stay is usually no more than two weeks. The number of these beds has fluctuated since the 1970s, due largely to the changing financial incentives set up by policy and regulatory agencies. I was practicing in the Washington, DC area in 1974, when insurance companies commonly began to require preauthorization for both outpatient therapies and inpatient stays, leading to the gradual decrease in the length of stay for any one hospitalization.

Contrast that with the usual minimum of three months for inpatients during my residency at the University of Virginia Hospital. Back then patients with federal insurance were sometimes covered for an entire year of inpatient care for psychiatric treatment. They also had a major medical supplement of

$50,000 per patient per lifetime for catastrophic coverage or for treatment of difficult-to-treat medical conditions, including psychiatric treatment. This allowed for intensive inpatient and outpatient treatments for patients with serious psychiatric illnesses. And in case $50,000 seems ridiculously low to your modern ears, the daily cost of a private room on the psychiatric unit at the University of Virginia Hospital was $44 in those days. A semi-private room was $42, and a bed in one of the four-bed wards was $40 per day. Outpatient appointments were in the range of $30 to $35 per session. So $50,000 could buy a lot of care in those days.

We had several patients who were hospitalized for over one year, necessary because they were in intensive psychoanalytic psychotherapy, with or without medication management, and were at risk for self-harm at very stressful times during their therapy. This also allowed them to focus on their therapy without having to deal with the demands and stresses of daily life.

There were a number of private hospitals that had originally been established to care for patients who could afford to pay out of pocket for their treatment, and these hospitals had begun to also treat patients who were dependent on insurance for payment of the costs of their treatment. Chestnut Lodge in Rockville, Maryland was one of these hospitals. It is the hospital that treated the woman who wrote the exceptional book *I Never Promised You A Rose Garden*, based on her treatment there with a well-known therapist. Shepphard and Enoch Pratt was another hospital in Towson, Maryland that also treated these severely ill psychiatric patients. McLean Hospital in Boston, Massachusetts was another such hospital.

Chestnut Lodge was closed many years ago due to the increasing restrictions on inpatient lengths of stay. Most of these hospitals have been closed or converted to acute care units. There was also access to specialized care in many of these hospitals, such as for individuals with severe eating disorders. Most all of those specialized units have been closed down. I have learned that Shepphard-Pratt and McLean Hospital have recently reopened units for the long term treatment of patients who can afford to pay for their care without utilizing insurance benefits.

This brings us to the heart of the current dilemma. With the lack of available inpatient treatment wards, this very vulnerable population of chronically ill psychiatric patients and profoundly mentally retarded children has been unable to receive adequate psychiatric treatment. These individuals will never have the capacity to be autonomous and independent. They do best in a protected, structured, nurturing and low-stimulus environment such as that provided by the old long-term state hospitals. This is the most ethical and humane treatment for these very psychologically and neurodevelopmentally damaged human beings.

Because the actual costs of the care of these people are currently less obvious than the costs of maintaining the long-term hospitals they need, there is still a lot of resistance to considering a transition back to this older form of treatment. Since many of the costs are borne by the correctional systems, they will not readily show up on economic reports of the overall costs of delivering psychiatric care at the present time. Also the human costs of being incarcerated are substantial for these individuals. The costs related to the homelessness of many of these persons also would not show up on most of the economic measurements. Dr. Sisti's group is to be commended for bringing this issue to the forefront of psychiatric thinking and planning for the future care of these patients.

So we must look at the economic issues underlying the current system of care and the costs of transiting back to the older asylum system. While I have been formally trained as a physician and psychiatrist, I have also endeavored to read extensively about economic issues over the past 35 to 40 years, generally with an emphasis on Austrian economics. I guess you could say I have an informal minor in economics.

I do not think we can intelligently think through these issues without looking at the economics of the nation at large. Much of my information has come from newsletters that looked at the fundamentals underlying the economic system, most with a primary focus on investment. Nevertheless, they also provided an ongoing look at the changing trends in the national economy. The writers that I consider the most relevant to my own concerns currently are James Dale Davidson of *Strategic Investment*, David Stockman of *David Stockman's Contra Corner* and *Gary North's Specific Questions*. All of these can be accessed online. North and Davidson are subscription sites.

As a nation we have been facing a difficult transition from an expanding economy to a more fragile, unrealistic 'pseudo expanding' economy. This has been taking place during the past 15 years, since the recession that followed the dot-com bubble of the late 1990s. The recession of 2008-2009 was the most obvious and significant effect. The Federal Reserve bailed out the big banks and American International Group (AIG) and nationalized the mortgage agencies, Fannie Mae and Freddie Mac, to prevent a catastrophic meltdown of the economy. This has created enormous deficits in the national budget, over one trillion dollars annually for several fiscal years. The total of the on- and off-budget federal debt plus the present cost of the entitlements of Social Security, Medicare and Medicaid are somewhere above two hundred trillion dollars and climbing. This greatly exceeds the amount not only of the GDP of the American economy but also of the *global* economy, making it completely unsustainable. Most of this debt will be defaulted on, wiping out a significant amount of digital wealth and bankrupting some large financial corporations, among others. This will liquidate a lot of the high-risk debt in the system, eventually allowing for a return to a more appropriate use of debt in financially rational ways. But the initial fallout will take down responsible companies, who are dependent on the status quo of the current system, in addition to the irresponsible central banks, large financial institutions and corporations that have benefited from this unrealistic system.

This current system cannot last much longer and cannot be depended upon to provide reliably for these long term patients who will require care for many decades. The large healthcare systems in this region have all taken on enormous debt to build as least five new state-of-the-art hospitals within the past two decades. None of them are making an adequate profit that will realistically allow them to service their debt.

One of the criticisms leveled at the old asylums was that they deprived patients of privacy and maintained them in large wards that just covered the basics, a roof over their heads, three meals a day, heat in the cold weather and clothing that consisted of hospital gowns or hand-me-downs other people had discarded. Most people who did not have professional experience with these settings were horrified by these conditions. What they could not see was that the patients were safe and their routines were structured for them. If one spends his or her days mostly rocking in a rocking chair staring out into space, it is nice to be left alone without more being asked of you. Building a state of the art hospital would be wasted on these patients. It would fail to address their most basic need for a low stimulus environment that provides safety, medication, food, a bed to sleep in and no expectations. For those patients who are somewhat higher functioning, there could be activities they could take part in that are part of the basic functioning of the hospital community. A fancy facility is overkill for this.

I had the experience of spending some time with one of these patients when I was a resident. This was a woman in her early to mid-thirties, who had spent several years in one of the state hospitals in our region. She had been attempting to transition into community care and had been living with an aunt and uncle who were very supportive. Nevertheless she was in the psychiatric unit because of suicidal impulses and the fear that she would not be able to manage life outside the long-term hospital. I was on call one night when she was pacing the hall, unable to sleep because she was very anxious. The nurse asked me to see her, and I talked with her at some length. She told me that she had spent nine months in a catatonic state, completely bedfast and with a feeding tube in her nose down into her stomach. She had vivid memories about that time and reported feeling very secure with her caregivers during that time. She had continued to have hallucinations during the time she was catatonic. Several different medicines were tried before she received one that began to lessen the intensity of her hallucinations. By the end of the nine months, she began to come out of the catatonic state. She had gradually improved, to the point that she was active on the unit and eventually was able to work in the garden on the grounds. As she improved she decided that she wanted to return to her family and her aunt and uncle were happy to have her come live with them again.

But even with the support of her family, she found it much harder to transition back into the community than she had expected She was beginning to feel like she was a failure. Her hallucinations were still intermittently present and had become more intense since she left the state hospital. Toward the end of the time I spent with her, I asked her about the time she was catatonic. She could remember feeling that she could not do anything for herself. She was overwhelmed by her hallucinations and just gave up any attempt to care for herself. I asked her why she did that, and she thought for several minutes before she answered. "I just needed that time," was what she said. She remained in the unit for several months, and she always smiled at me and greeted me when we saw each other in the hallway. She was not my patient, so I do not know if she was successful in her transition into the community. But she was clearly glad to see me and had benefitted from her time in the facility and being able to tell me her story.

I have always been grateful for the insight into what it was like for her in the long-term hospital, including the deep sense of security she had from her caregivers there. This was clearly an important part of the therapeutic experience for her, perhaps even as much so or more important than the medication she was prescribed. And it gave me a new respect for the needs these severely psychotic patients have, including the need for a calm, supportive and undemanding environment in which to live with their illness. Just enduring their psychosis is as much as most of them can handle. So they do not need, nor would they appreciate anything fancy. It is not necessary to provide anymore than the old asylums were providing. Building state-of-the-art hospitals is both unnecessary and financially risky. The old asylums had it right.

Chapter Six

Economic Constraints

Many communities, including the Tri-Cities area of northeast Tennessee and southwest Virginia, have never really recovered from the 2008-2009 recession, with little improvement in the local economies since that time. They have not returned to a reasonable post-recession expansion. The minimal expansion that may be claimed is due to the increase of debt in municipal bonds, many of which are unlikely to be repaid. This includes the building of three hospitals, with the closing of two of the community hospitals, and apparently none of the three have been able to earn a significant profit since opening in the past three or four years.

As a nation we are facing another recession by the end of this year or early in 2017. The stock market appears to be at an unrealistic high and very vulnerable to a significant drop in market indexes when overvalued stocks correct to the downside. This will occur in the context of a global recession, which is already evident in China and Europe. The commodities markets are already contracting with no evidence that they will reach a stable balance anytime soon.

President Obama's Affordable Care Act (ObamaCare), which was to be affordable, is anything but. Many families are paying high premiums for what is essentially only catastrophic coverage due to the very high deductibles that they have to pay out of pocket before their coverage kicks in. Many people have reported to me that they have had to take on even higher premiums with the start of 2016. And one person I know reports that her health insurer has already let her know that they are attempting to get another 30% to 40 % increase in her premium for 2017. It's no wonder that having this insurance has had to be coerced by the punitive tax on the uninsured. As if protecting one's family with a health insurance policy is not motive enough for most people.

Many states are struggling to cover their current expenses, and robbing their already underfunded pension funds are the short-term solution for that. Detroit is the first major city to bankrupt out of their pension responsibilities and other unmanageable debts, but it is not likely to be the last.

All of this will inevitably mean less funds to provide new treatment programs or for the building of new asylums. Particularly in the case of a return to the older asylum system, the funds are not likely to be available for major new building projects. And given that the population has nearly doubled since the mid-1950s, the number of long-term psychiatric beds that would be needed is likely to be at a minimum, around 500,000 to 600,000. This would include the almost 320,000 seriously mentally ill prisoners incarcerated in the correctional system (Torrey, et al., 2010). It would also include the 20 to 25% of the homeless population with some form of severe mental illness (*National Coalition for the Homeless*, 2009).

So what do we do? I have given this a lot of thought over the years. I do not think new building projects are a realistic option. However, there are some alternatives to new building projects that would be reasonable to consider. I think a return to open wards for the delivery of medical care generally, including psychiatric care, would be a move in the right direction. The new hospitals that have been built in the past two decades have generally provided private rooms for every patient except for the beds in ICUs and Critical Care units where the beds are open to the nursing station with some kind of barrier between patient areas.

The regular patient rooms have created significant isolation for many patients. The hospital floors are generally understaffed, and patients may only see someone on the nursing staff at the change of shift and when medications are dispensed. If the patient doesn't have someone like a family member to get assistance for him or her, he/she may have a long wait to get the attention of a staff member. I do not believe this has been in best interests of the patients.

On an open ward, the nursing station is generally located somewhere in the unit itself. That allows the nurses to continually observe patients and address their needs or concerns very quickly. This was the standard of care at the State University of Iowa Hospital where I did a rotating internship before starting my psychiatry residency. I was able to observe the effectiveness of the care on these units. I have been sad to see the move to all private rooms because of the isolation of the patients this system requires. Additionally, the support of the other patients on an open unit can be a very therapeutic part of the hospital experience. And the ward system would appear to be much more cost effective than the system we have now.

There would also need to be some private or semi-private rooms available on each unit for special situations that required that kind of isolation, such as patients undergoing treatment that causes significant immune suppression. On one of my surgery rotations during my internship in Iowa there was a 14-bed burn unit that was separate from the open ward. That unit was a mix of private, two and four bed rooms. That mix of ward beds and beds with more privacy worked very well for the patients and the medical and nursing staff on that unit.

A second consideration regarding a return to the old asylum system has to do with the size and location of the institutions. When these hospitals were first built, they were usually large institutions that served as treatment centers for large regions of the state they were in. During medical school and residency I became somewhat familiar with the state hospitals in Virginia. There were four hospitals for chronic psychiatric patients. Eastern State Hospital in Williamsburg was the first hospital for the mentally ill in the nation. It was established in the late 1700s. Central State Hospital in Petersburg was the first hospital established to take mentally ill African-Americans, most of whom were slaves. This started in the 1850s prior to the Civil War. Western

State Hospital in Staunton served the needs of the western and northern counties in the state. Southwestern State Hospital in Marion, the most recently established, served the needs of all the counties west and south of Roanoke. All these facilities are primarily acute and subacute treatment hospitals now with lengths of stay in the two to three month range. Many of the older buildings at Southwestern State Hospital have been torn down, and a new building to serve 177 patients was completed in early 1990. The building that housed the criminally insane was taken over by the Virginia Department of Corrections in 1981. It is used for inpatient care for inmates of the Virginia prison system.

The Lynchburg Colony in Lynchburg was established initially for the care of epileptics in 1910. In 1914 it took on the care of those who were profoundly mentally retarded as well. These patients usually spent their entire lives in the institution. In 1983 the name was changed to the Central Virginia Training Center. Today it remains the largest of the five Commonwealth facilities caring for individuals with mental retardation. These facilities are currently in the process of being shut down, and this is reported to be happening at a much faster pace than occurred with the shutting down of the long-term beds for the chronically mentally ill.

Most of the patients treated in these long-term institutions were from counties or cities at some distance from the hospital. Once the patients had been there for several years, most of them no longer had contact with their families. The institution had become home to them. Families went on with their lives without the patient. The distances required for travel placed a burden on the family that eventually outweighed their sense of responsibility to visit someone who might not even respond to them. So the institutions provided for the care of these patients without involvement with the families for the most part.

Currently, it would not be unreasonable to consider smaller institutions that could serve a smaller number of counties. Travel distances are no longer as much of an issue so it would be easier for families, to remain in contact with their institutionalized family members. But this would be unlikely to lead to the patient's being discharged from the hospital if they remained chronically psychotic and failed to respond to treatment. This would be the case for profoundly retarded or brain-injured patients as well. The institution would remain the primary care agent for these individuals under those circumstances.

I have one last suggestion for providing appropriate buildings for these institutions. There should be an exploration of older buildings within the geographic area where the institution is to be placed, looking for buildings that could be renovated to provide the necessary space for the housing of these individuals. As has been previously discussed, most of these patients are largely indifferent to their surroundings as long as they feel safe and cared for by an attentive staff, so the facility does not have to have a particular look, age or style.

The first place to look would be the Asylum Projects at www.asylumprojects.org, which has a listing of all the old asylums and their current status. This is one of the Wikipedia projects but you cannot access it through Wikipedia, only through their website. While many of the older buildings were torn down years ago, some of these buildings are still standing. The Asylum Projects is trying to save some of the remaining buildings as historically important. It is possible that a number of them might be workable, with renovation, to be returned to their original function in the mental health system.

There may also be unused commercial space that could be converted to a combination of open wards and smaller, more private rooms for higher functioning patients. These may be more readily available in areas that have suffered more economically in recent decades.

Another possibility would be failed colleges with campuses that would be suitable for use as asylums. For instance, there have been two colleges that closed in Bristol, Virginia within recent decades, and both have reasonably large campuses that are currently largely unused. One closed in 1976, but part of the campus was used for a private school for children from kindergarten through eighth grade. The school was there from 1976 through 1999, at which point they relocated to a new campus. Most of the buildings are not used at this time.

The second college closed much more recently (2014) due to financial difficulties and loss of accreditation. Those buildings are currently unused. Failed institutions like these may be very appropriate for the kinds of units that would work for the long-term care of these vulnerable individuals. They would likely have a mix of buildings that could utilize the open ward model for some patients and semi-private rooms for patients who were capable of a higher level of self-care.

There are also a number of churches that have closed that might also have appropriate facilities for providing such care. They do not have the same amount of space that the college campuses have, but smaller institutions would likely be viable in a number of areas with less population density. For instance a moderate sized church, with a separate building that housed a daycare center, recently closed in Bristol, Tennessee. Older public school buildings that have been closed might offer another option.

The last thing to keep in mind is that these patients are not likely to improve enough to be able to maintain themselves outside a hospital setting. If the decision were to be made to transition back to the asylum model for the long-term care of these patients, it would need to be funded as an ongoing annual cost to the state and/or the local counties served.

On the positive side, there would be significant savings for the state correctional systems if these patients were in the more appropriate setting of a long-term psychiatric facility. Additionally, the costs of care for the homeless, who mostly access care through emergency rooms and brief inpatient hospitalizations, should also be less with the more stable and safe units in the asylum. And the local communities would be safer if the more paranoid and potentially violent persons in this group were safely maintained in the long-term hospital setting.

Relying on the use of high levels of debt to finance new building projects appears to me to be a high-risk way to provide for these patients. It is unlikely to be sustainable over the long term. We do not need additional expensive failed institutions. Going back to a state or county-funded simpler system for delivering care to these patients would appear to be a better approach. It would also be more financially sound going forward.

Chapter Seven

Final Thoughts

I am very aware that the process of transitioning back to an asylum model of care for the chronically mentally ill will be a difficult and demanding undertaking. And I am not naive enough to believe that it will be accomplished in a short time. The current model of care for these patients, as inadequate as it is, will remain with us for some time to come. It is part of the present *status quo* that is coming under increasing levels of stress in the face of economic crises, shortages of critical natural resources, environmental damage from industrial sources and the increasing climate instability. It is important to begin to explore this issue in order to develop realistic plans for the long-term care of some of our most vulnerable individuals.

I believe it would be important to open an on going discussion with Dr. Sisti's team, since they have obviously done a lot of research on this very challenging problem. I believe they could be of assistance in developing the early models for the transition. E. Fuller Torrey's *Treatment Advocacy Center* would likely be another good source for ideas for these changes. The core issue comes down to how we are to provide care for people who will, for the most part, be unable to be productive citizens within our society. This is not a situation that lends itself to profit-making solutions, which makes it a poor fit in this economy. Finding the funding to begin the first steps in the process will be very difficult and may require government grants for the first, somewhat experimental programs. This could also be something that some of the large foundations would be willing to contribute to. Another possibility could be funding from the correctional system tied into plans to admit some of the mentally ill inmates to pilot asylum programs. This would relieve the prisons and jails of the extra expenses they have for these inmates. Every effort should be made to keep the costs down by providing basic services to these individuals in a safe, low-stimulus, no-frills environment. It is likely that current rules and regulations that govern healthcare facilities will need to be revised to allow for these programs to operate as economically as possible.

Recently I have been reading an important book that explores the issues we face in order to survive the climate changes that we share some responsibility for. It is titled *The End of the Long Summer: Why We Must Remake Our Civilization to Survive on a Volatile Earth*, published in 2009. The author is Dianne Dumanoski, and she is an environmental journalist who has written extensively on these issues over the past 30 years. She is primarily focused on the topics of climate change and the destructiveness of the human enterprise since the advent of the Industrial Revolution. She reports on a number of local, regional and international activist groups that are trying to promote positive change in addressing the transitions that need to take place economically and socially if we are to avoid the worst outcomes. I can highly recommend it for anyone interested in becoming more educated about these larger issues.

I view the issue of asylums as being one aspect of the larger issue of how we prepare for a difficult and challenging future. The current lack of realistic planning for these vulnerable individuals appears to be an abandonment. It would be tragic if this type of neglect continues to be a characteristic of our culture and would not bode well for us in the long run. Medicine has become dominated by large corporations and government bureaucracies over the 50 years since I graduated from medical school. And a lot of the art of medicine is being lost to economic decisions that have lost sight of the needs of patients and of their providers.

As Dumanoski points out in her book, the economic historian Karl Polanyi has aptly noted that human society has become "an accessory of the economic system" of the modern western culture. Human beings should not be treated as afterthoughts, and the future of humanity should not be left to markets to decide. We need to thoughtfully and intentionally plan for an uncertain future, and we had best begin immediately.

Bibliography

Buckley, Peter F.; Miller, Brian J.; Lehrer, Douglas S.; Castle, David J.,
    Psychiatric Comorbidities and   Schizophrenia, *Schizophrenia
    Bulletin* **35** (2), 383-402, (2009).

Department of Health and Human Services, Nursing Home Data
    Compendium, 2013.

James, Doris; Glaze, Lauren, Mental Health Problems of Prison and Jail
    Inmates, *Bureau of Justice Statistics Special Report*, September 2006,
    revised December 14, 2006.

Dumanoski, Dianne, *The End of the Long Summer: Why We Must Remake
    Our Civilization to Survive on a Volatile Earth*, 2009.

National Coalition for the Homeless, Mental Illness and Homelessness, July,
    2009

Sisti, Dominic A.; Segal, Andrea G.; Emanuel, Ezekiel J., Improving Long-
    Term Psychiatric Care: Bring Back the Asylum, *Journal of the
    American Medical Association (JAMA)* **313** (3), 243-244, January 20,
    2015.

The Associated Press, Nursing homes turn to eviction to drop difficult
    patients, *Bristol Herald Courier,* A1, A9, May 9, 2016.

Torrey, E. Fuller; Kennard, Aaron D.; Eslinger, Don; Lamb, Richard; Pavle,
    James (May 2010). More Mentally Ill Persons Are in Jails and
    Prisons Than Hospitals: A Survey of the States. Arlington, Virginia:
    Treatment Advocacy Center. Pp. 1-22.

U.S. Department of Justice, Office of Justice Programs, Bureau of Justice
    Statistics, 2014.

About the Author

Linda R. Thompson graduated from the University of Virginia School of Medicine in 1966, and did a rotating internship at the State University of Iowa Hospital in 1966-1967, before returning to the University of Virginia Hospital for her residency in psychiatry from 1967-1971. She then entered psychoanalytic training at the Washington Psychoanalytic Institute in 1972, completing the training and graduating in 1983. She maintained a general psychiatric practice in the Tri-Cities area of northeast Tennessee and southwest Virginia from 1984 through 2014. She continues to maintain a small part-time psychotherapy practice. She is now devoting most of her time to writing, and her next book reviewing her medical education is pending.

www.ingramcontent.com/pod-product-compliance
Lightning Source LLC
Chambersburg PA
CBHW070408190526
45169CB00003B/1167